T0116290

Hair Color at Home

What to Buy and How to Apply

Beautiful Hair Color at Home

by C. A. Beebe

Order this book online at www.trafford.com
or email orders@trafford.com

Most Trafford titles are also available at major online book retailers.

Printed in Victoria, BC, Canada.

ISBN: 978-1-4120-4233-8 (Soft)

*Our mission is to efficiently provide the world's finest, most comprehensive
book publishing service, enabling every author to experience success.
To find out how to publish your book, your way, and have it available
worldwide, visit us online at www.trafford.com*

Trafford rev. 11/25/2009

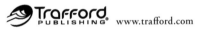 www.trafford.com

North America & international
toll-free: 1 888 232 4444 (USA & Canada)
phone: 250 383 6864 ♦ fax: 812 355 4082

WARNING - DISCLAIMER

This book is designed to provide basic information on the use of hair color at home. It is a general guide and not intended to be used in place of manufacturers' instructions. Always follow manufacturers' instructions.

Every effort was made to make this guide as accurate as possible. The author and publisher shall have neither liability nor responsibility for any hair color attempted at home.

The information contained in this book is also not to be used to perform cosmetology services without a license or for compensation.

Acknowledgements

My friend Deb can solve almost any problem. When I asked if she knew anyone who could help prepare this hair color information for printing, she introduced me to Jim Hatch. He edited the copy, insisted on the glossary, did page layout and formatted the book for printing. He also now knows more about violet than he ever intended, but without him I might never have gotten this book into print. I owe him many thanks. And thanks to Deb for always knowing who to go to for help.

Cheryl Beebe

Contents

Introduction

Several years ago I read that 36 million women and men did home hair color. That number has likely increased substantially. Are you one of those millions? Are you always confident that when you buy a box of home color the results will be pleasing? If you have doubts or questions, this book is for you.

Coloring hair is more complicated than choosing a picture on a box in the color aisle at Walmart. I hope *Hair Color at Home* will teach you the basics of color so you can knowledgeably choose the color product that will give you the results you seek. In addition to correct color selection, you will learn some application secrets that will help you achieve better results.

The beauty salon industry would prefer you receive all color services in a salon with a licensed cosmetologist. Truthfully, there are many color services you probably shouldn't attempt at home. My hope is that if you do plan to color your hair at home, you will get the best possible results.

This book is the result of years of observing clients who were coloring at home and were not happy with the outcome. As I tried to find resources to help them, I found that there was very little published guidance materials for customers faced with selection of the right product. You could make a guess, but if you guessed wrong *everyone* was going to notice.

This book will bridge that gap. When you grasp this knowledge you will be able to purchase and apply home hair color products with much more confidence. The result will be beautiful, healthy hair.

Now, let's get started.

Chapter 1
Why should I color my hair?

We have all heard the phrase "the grass is greener." The adventure of change is probably the biggest reason for altering hair color. We want what we don't have.

There are also many reasons for choosing to do the hair color at home. With our current economy, the number one reason for coloring hair at home is the cost savings, but lack of time and the convenience of a box at home are also factors. Whether we choose coloring at home or in a salon, let's examine the benefits of colored hair.

Fine hair
If you have fine hair, artificial color can give your hair body. Many color products swell the hair giving the feeling of having more hair, which is great for a fine head of hair.

Coarse hair
If you have coarse hair, color can make the hair more pliable and easier to style. In a sense, it softens the coarseness.

Normal hair
The remaining reasons to color hair are mainly for the appearance. Color can make you look younger. Some say it is the most inexpensive way to take off ten years. Color can cover or blend gray. It can boost morale by giving you a new look and can add fun and excitement to your life. Changing your hair color drastically

makes a statement and can definitely get you noticed. A new color can also be as subtle as a slight lightening or brightening.

What are my choices if I decide to color my hair?

There are three main options for hair color at home or in the salon. These are *temporary, semi-permanent and permanent color.* As color has become more advanced, these three types have been expanded into colors that fit in between the categories. This somewhat blurs the lines. One currently popular choice is demi-permanent. It is longer lasting than semi-permanent but not as lasting as permanent. However, for the purpose of this book we are sticking to the original three categories with only a slight mention of some of the in-between categories. Let's begin by discussing temporary color.

> *New hair color is the fastest way to take 10 years off your age.*

Temporary

Temporary color is sometimes known as "no commitment" color. It is generally considered a color that washes out from shampoo to shampoo. Some temporary color can last a couple of shampoos, particularly if it is used often or on porous hair. (More about hair porosity in Chapter 2.) Temporary color has no power to lighten hair. It can change the tone of hair or can make hair appear darker. It is often used to blend in gray or to temporarily refresh faded hair color between permanent color services. It has no alcohol, peroxide or ammonia and requires no mixing. It can be used immediately after a perm or relaxer.

There are several types of temporary color products available in drug and big box stores. Some examples are color shampoos, colored foams (otherwise known as color mousse), and liquid color such as Fanciful Rinse. Recently, colored gels have made a strong showing especially with the younger crowd. Other options for temporary color are sprays and glitter sprays. These are usually for theatrical or party hair. My town has a big St. Patty's day parade every year and often even dogs and horses are wearing green temporary color spray in the parade. Color shampoo is used as a substitute for your normal shampoo but the foams and liquids are designed to be applied to clean, towel dried hair. You can apply gels, sprays and glitter to the entire head or single out specific areas for application. Some temporary color can be made semi-permanent by adding heat.

CAUTION: *Many very bright colors are available as temporary color. They look great accenting dark hair but can be shocking or fluorescent on light hair. They can also grab and hold on porous hair, especially bleached and frosted hair.*

Semi-permanent

Semi-permanent color is color with some commitment. It is also known as "deposit-only color." It's designed to last for six or more shampoos. Semi-permanent color generally does not penetrate the hair strand. It coats and deposits color only and it has no lightening ability. However, some semi-permanents may have an activating solution (you mix two bottles together), giving it the potential to slightly lighten some hair.

The day you apply the color to the hair is the deepest (darkest) the hair will be. The color then fades with each subsequent shampoo. The name semi-permanent implies that eventually all the color will be gone, but many times you can see the remains of semi-permanent color for a very long time, particularly if you have used the color repeatedly. Sometimes the semi-permanent color can only be eliminated by cutting it off.

CAUTION: *Many manufacturers recommend that you apply semi-permanent color to the entire head. However, if the previous color application has not faded from the ends and/or the ends have become porous, the current color may process faster and darker in the ends.* This is, in my opinion, the main trouble with semi-permanent color. You can overcome this tendency by putting the color in the new growth first and only applying color to the ends later if needed.

Semi-permanent color is great for blending hair that has up to 50% gray. The hair that is not gray doesn't have to change significantly, but the white/gray hairs can be covered and this will give a younger look. With the hair color fading gradually, the hair tends not to have the strong line of demarcation (the line separating new hair growth and colored hair). You can choose to color once, let it fade away and never color again, or you can also continue to color whenever you wish.

Some semi-permanent hair colors can be used immediately after a chemical service. Always check the manufacturer's instructions to confirm whether or not you can use a particular semi-permanent color after perms or relaxers.

Permanent color
Permanent hair color is color with maximum commitment. It is designed to be on the hair, or at least have some of the effects of color on the hair, until it is cut off. Permanent color can darken hair, lighten hair, and is best for covering gray. Bleach is also in the category of permanent hair color. Permanent colors usually come in a liquid or creme form that is mixed with some type of developer, usually peroxide. The two solutions mixed together cause a chemical reaction. This reaction allows the color to penetrate inside the hair and deposit color or lift color from inside the hair. Permanent color can deposit color and lighten in one step. As the molecules penetrate inside the hair, they grow and lodge (get stuck) inside the hair strand. There is also some color staining happening. After the required amount of time (as per instructions), you shampoo and rinse the remaining color. The color that stays in the hair is said to be permanent even though it can fade with shampooing, sun and other fade factors.

It is generally recommended that you wait at least a week between permanent color and any other chemical service. If you are a weekly salon client, do not color for a week plus one shampoo after a perm or relaxer to ensure maximum results from both services. In other words, weekly clients should wait two weeks to color their hair with permanent color after any other chemical service.

Keep in mind that some delicate hair is not strong enough to be both permed or relaxed and colored with permanent color. If your hair is somewhat fragile, you may not be able to do both. Even the strongest hair may need to be reconditioned with a protein conditioner to withstand both

> *Don't forget to reconition colored hair. Also use products to protect your new color from sun and fading.*

chemical services. Also be aware that perming after a color can cause major fading. If you decide to do both, always perm first if you are deepening your color. If you are lightening your hair, it may not matter which process is done first.

Keep in mind that coloring even several weeks after a perm can cause curl relaxation. My advice for clients that color is to be sure to condition to protect your hair. If you perm and color, make sure to recondition (strengthen) regularly to keep your hair in great shape.

Demi-permanent color
A quick mention of demi-permanent color is in order here. It cannot lighten hair but is generally designed to last longer than semi-permanent colors. You would treat color selection and application of a demi color in the same way you would choose a semi-permanent.

Color options
Deciding which of the three types of color (temporary, semi-permanent, or permanent) you need to use cannot be done until you decide what outcome you need. The three basic options are:

1. Going lighter

2. Going darker

3. Staying the same level of darkness but changing tone

Let's briefly discuss each option.

Lightening
The only way hair can be lightened is with permanent color or bleach. If this is your desired outcome, don't even think about looking at boxes of semi-permanent or temporary color.

Deepening
If your choice is to go darker with your hair color, you may choose permanent, semi-permanent or temporary color. If you have significant gray to cover, the best choice for darkening is permanent color. If you have only a little gray and would just like to blend and/or camouflage this gray, semi-permanent color may be your best option. This is particularly true if you are just beginning to experiment with coloring your hair. If all you want is darker hair for a day or two, use temporary color.

Changing tone
You may change your tone with any of the three color types just like the instructions for deepening color. Going from brown to red is probably best done originally with semi-permanent color. If you don't like the change, it takes less time for the color to fade back to your natural color. If your goal is to make gray or white hair look less yellow or brighter and whiter, temporary color works just great. *If it's an experiment, use temporary or semi-permanent color.*

Technique options
Professional colorists have many techniques such as foiling, frosting, tipping or scrunching at their disposal to give clients whatever effect they request. The experienced home colorist may also learn and master some advanced techniques. However, for the purpose of this book, we are concentrating on the basics. The two main techniques or applications available to the home colorist are a solid color or a dimensional color, frost, for example. These are both readily available in the color aisle of most retail stores.

Solid color

A solid color is applied to the entire head. The goal is usually to have the color look the same from scalp to ends. Most natural hair is slightly lighter on the ends and you may prefer this look for your hair coloring. This is especially true if you have long hair. If your goal is natural looking hair color, you never want your ends to be darker than the hair next to the scalp. When we discuss application techniques, we will talk about how to get the best results when your desired outcome is a solid color.

Dimensional color

Frosts and weaves (foil highlights) are examples of dimensional color. What this really means is that all the hair is not the same color. Some hairs could be blonde and some brown or any number of other color choices. Dimensional color could also mean that the hair in the nape is dark and the hair originating from the crown is light. Dimensional color can be thin streaks or thick chunks. As many colors as you desire are possible. Dimensional color remains popular regardless of trends because the line of demarcation (where the colored hair meets the natural hair) is usually less noticeable than with a solid color. This means that the upkeep can be less frequent. Current fashions often dictate what the popular looks are for dimensional color. It may be subtle or it may be bold, even garish. Watching television and looking at fashion magazines will show you the newest trends.

Closing thoughts

Hair color is fun. The change it brings can be uplifting, and being pampered is awesome. If you want to be pampered, find a professional stylist to color your hair. Use the knowledge you gain from this book to better discuss your options with your stylist. If you have knowledge of temporary, semi-permanent and permanent color, you can make informed choices. The same is true about the decision to have a solid color or a dimensional color. Knowledge is power and this book can make you a very educated salon customer.

However, if a salon is out of the question and you want to achieve fantastic hair color at home, this book can help you reach that goal. Regardless of whether your hair color is to be done at home or in a salon, keep reading. There is a lot more to learn so you can do great hair color at home.

Hair Color Horror Story

I was in the color aisle at Walmart when I heard a grandma and her teenage granddaughter arguing about how to fix the girl's accidentally produced flaming orange hair.

It was then that I knew I had to write this book.

Chapter 2
All about hair

We are going to start this chapter talking about hair. Giving you a thorough understanding of hair and the ability to analyze and categorize your own hair will be the goal of this chapter. At the end of this chapter you will be able to answer fundamental questions that will lead to a successful hair color experience. The first question we will address is "What kind of hair do I have?" This question requires us to consider the four main characteristics of hair: density, texture, porosity and color.

Density

The definition of hair density is the number of hairs per square inch of scalp. This characteristic has the least effect of the four in achieving our goal of beautiful home hair color. Still, it does count significantly when doing dimensional hair color. If you have a very thick head of hair that has been frosted or highlighted, you have to have more hairs colored to be noticeable. If your hair is thin or sparse and you have lightened a lot of hair, the color could look almost like a solid color. Also, if you have thick hair you must have enough product to entirely cover all of the hair being colored. If your hair is thick and long, you may need to buy two boxes of color to have what you need for complete coverage. So, density counts but it is the least important of the four characteristics of hair.

Now, analyze your density. Is your hair thick, thin or average? If you don't already know, ask your friends' permission to let you run your fingers through their hair and compare the amount of hair they have with yours. Can you figure out your density? If you can, great. If you are having trouble, ask for help from family and friends.

Texture

Fine hair appears to take color darker than coarse hair.

Hair texture is determined by how fat or thin each individual hair is. Do you have skinny hair? If you do, we call it fine hair. If each strand of hair has a pretty big circumference, we call it coarse hair. The hair that is neither skinny nor fat is considered to have medium texture. If you are using permanent color (the color that penetrates) on fine hair, there is less space inside the hair strand for the color. The color then has to bunch up. Squishing those color molecules together makes the hair look darker. Therefore, if you use permanent color on fine hair, you will want to choose a lighter color.

The opposite is true for very coarse hair. The color molecules have a big space to fill and may look lighter because the gaps aren't filled. This can be remedied by using a darker color when coloring coarse hair. Medium texture generally causes no problems.

This is a simplistic explanation of chemical processes, but the moral of the story is if you have fine hair, choose a lighter color than your desired shade. If you have coarse hair you may have to choose a darker color to achieve your desired shade. My best advice for coarse hair is to choose the target shade first. You can always go darker later.

What is your texture? Is it fine, medium or coarse? If you don't know, ask friends for help. Pull out one hair and have several friends do the same. Compare the girth between your hair and the other hairs. Can you see some differences? Do you know your texture? If you do, we can keep moving forward. If you still can't tell, ask your hair stylist. Remember that as you age and your hair starts to gray, the texture may change.

Porosity

When we talk about porosity we are talking about the hair's ability to absorb. Porous hair is likely damaged hair. What this means for hair color is that if your hair is very porous, it will absorb color very quickly. It also loses color very quickly. Porous hair does not give you long-lasting color. It fades. If the hair at the ends is porous (damaged) but the hair close to your scalp is normal, the color will process differently on the hair strand. The ends will be ready to rinse before the undamaged hair. If you only test the color on the ends and see that it is ready to rinse, the color at the scalp may not have processed long enough. In this case, porosity will determine your application technique and the timing.

Resistant hair does not absorb easily. It is nonporous hair and sometimes we call it stubborn hair. Resistant hair may require longer color timing. An example of resistant or nonporous hair could be the coarse gray hair on the temples or at the sideburn area.

How porous or damaged is your hair? Hair that is not in good condition should not be colored until you have restored some of the health through reconditioning. If you can't tell whether your hair is damaged just by the look and feel, pull your thumb and forefinger from the ends to scalp on a small section of hair. If your fingers slide right to the scalp, you are in good shape. If the hair ruffles as you stroke, you may have a porosity problem. If you have damage, fix the problem before you color. If the damage is minimal, apply the color to the normal hair first and to the porous hair after partial processing. The more porous the hair, the faster it absorbs.

Now you are ready to go to the last and most important characteristic of hair.

Color

We all have labels or names given to our hair color. The names are simple: gray, white, black, brown, blonde and red. Hair color companies generally label colors using Levels 1 to 10, Level 1 being the darkest.

Level 1 - Blue black

Level 2 - Black

Level 3 - Very dark brown

Level 4 - Dark brown

Level 5 - Medium brown

Level 6 - Light brown

Level 7 - Dark blonde

Level 8 - Medium blonde

Level 9 - Light blonde

Level 10 - Very light blonde or lightest blonde

Some companies vary slightly with the names, but this scale is as close to standard as I have found. For the purpose of explanation we will refer to white hair as Level 11. In reality white hair is hair without any pigment or color. Gray hair is a mixture of white hairs with brown or blonde hairs. Gray hair can be single strands that have started to lose pigment but still have a small amount left. What appears to us as gray hair is really a combination of white and pigmented hair. When we see the big picture, the whole head, we see gray hair. Keep in mind that for hair color purposes, the big picture is far more important than the color of individual strands. However, for formulating color the individual strands do count.

The United States is a melting pot of nationalities. Americans of primarily European heritage tend to have Level 4 through

Level 7 or 8 hair. The cultures that are most pure seem to have levels that are on the ends of the spectrum. Asians and Hispanics usually have hair between Level 1 and 3 or 4. Norwegians and those of Scandinavian descent mainly fall in the upper part of the spectrum with Levels 8 to 10. As for the world population, there are more people with black hair than any other color.

Find your level by comparing the names on the chart with your hair and by asking the opinion of others. I am sure you can come very close. Professionals have color swatches to be totally accurate and sometimes you will find color swatches in the color aisle to help. You must know your level, your starting place, as the first major component in the hair coloring process. Keep in mind that if you have gray hair, you have some white hairs (Level 11) and some hair of another level. For example, you can be a Level 5 (medium brown) with 10% Level 11 (white). Also, if you have longer hair, your level at the ends of your hair may be different than the level at the scalp. Make note of your level from scalp to ends.

In this section on color we must also comment on tone. A full discussion will come in the next chapter but for now you need to know that we categorize hair tone as warm or cool (ash). Gold, red and auburn are examples of the warm colors. Mousy or drab are names that characterize cool or ash colors. Dishwater blonde is another term you may have heard to describe ash hair color. Your color may also be neutral, neither warm nor cool. Make the determination of your tone now, either by sight or by comparison. The true importance of tone will be made clear in the chapter on lightening hair.

Do you know your level and tone?

Closing thoughts
This chapter focused on providing you with the information you will need to start the color process. You must analyze your hair

and answer the question "What type of hair do I have?" Your answer will include what you have determined about your hair's level and tone, porosity, texture and density. Don't proceed with coloring your hair until you have figured out this important information.

Chapter 3
The basics of color theory

To have a complete understanding of hair color you must start with basic knowledge of the color wheel. For those with an art background this is an easy chapter and you already know this information. If art wasn't your thing, stick with me because it is really important. The color wheel is the foundation for everything else we discuss in *Hair Color at Home*. It enables us to make our color selection and color selection is extremely important. Color theory is just as important as knowing your level. We must know the answer to the question, "What color do I want to be?" We learned levels in the last chapter and we will now learn about tones.

> *It's easier to learn this color information and do it right the first time than to try to fix your hair after a terrible accident.*

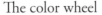

The color wheel

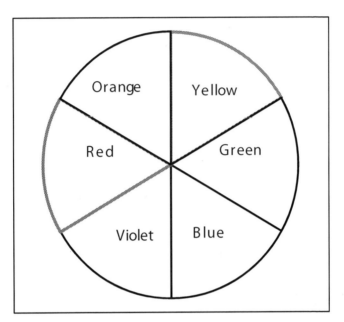

Primary colors are colors from which all others are made. Differing proportions of the primaries make every color we can see. There are three primaries. They are red, yellow and blue. Secondary colors are colors made by mixing two primary colors together. The secondary colors are orange, green and violet.

Blue + Yellow = Green

Yellow + Red = Orange

Red + Blue = Violet

The following may not be scientifically accurate but should help you visually understand hair and hair color and knowledge of the color wheel will help you understand tones.

Mostly we are concerned with warm or cool tones. We classify hair color or tone in three ways. Neutral is equal parts of primary colors. Ash or cool tones have more green, blue, or violet. Warm tones have more red, orange or yellow.

For hair coloring purposes natural looking hair is made with three parts yellow, two parts red and one part blue. Blue is the most dominant primary and yellow is the lightest. This combination gives a color that is neither warm nor cool, neither golden nor ash. With this combination the hair would be a neutral color. If you are talking about brown, it would be neutral brown.

If you add more blue you get into a darker shade, eventually getting to black or blue black, a Level 2 or 1.

When you lighten hair, the first molecule to leave the hair is blue. If you take out the blue, what is left? Two parts red and three parts yellow which is red-orange.

Red is the second molecule to leave the hair during the lightening process which means you get progressively lighter stages of orange until all the red is gone and then you have yellow.

If you continue to lighten, you can take the hair to pale yellow. If you lighten until the hair is white, no pigment left, you have hair that is probably damaged beyond redemption.

We can, however, make the hair appear white without taking out all the pigment. The way to cancel an unwanted color, in this case yellow, is to use a color on the color wheel that is directly across from the unwanted tone. If you have yellow hair and don't want it, use the opposing color, violet, to counteract or cancel the yellow. If we have orange hair and do not want orange, we would use a blue base color to counteract the orange. Finally if we have red hair and do not want the red we would use a color with a green base to eliminate the red. Conversely, if we have green hair (maybe from chlorine) we could use a red color to eliminate or camouflage the green.

This concept will save you a lot of experimentation: *If you have a color you don't want, use the opposing color on the color wheel to make it go away.*

Also remember: For the purpose of hair coloring, white hair has no pigment. No yellow. No red. No blue. To color white hair to look neutral, we must use more yellow than red and blue.

When you buy a hair color product, you can't always tell what the base is. If the information on the box doesn't indicate neutral or directly what the base color is, look for words like ash, warm or golden.

If we combine the information in Chapter 2 on levels with the information in Chapter 3 on tones we are ready to answer the second question of hair color: *What do I want to be?*

What level and what tone, either warm or cool, do you want for your final hair color outcome?

Once you have answered the first two questions—*What do I have? What do I want?* —you are ready to move on to the appropriate chapter.

Chapter 4 - Lightening hair with bleach

Chapter 5 - Lightening hair with color

Chapter 6 - Deepening your shade

Chapter 7 - Changing color while staying the same level

Closing thoughts

To many readers this chapter may be a review as they already know about color theory. To others it could be hard to understand. It is, however, critical information to give you full benefit from the next chapters. Reread this chapter or refer back to it as you continue your quest for great home hair color

Chapter 4
All about lightening hair with bleach

Lightening the hair is a popular choice with many home colorists. Although brunettes are a fast rising segment of the hair color market, blonde is usually the leader. The last statistic I read showed 39% of hair coloring done is an attempt to achieve blonde hair.

If your desire is to be a blonde, you must study this chapter to gain complete understanding. When you understand this chapter, you are over halfway to solving almost any hair color question.

There was a time when bleach was our only option for lightening hair. Since then we have discovered the use of colors to achieve lightened hair. Bleach is still a useful tool. This chapter, in fact, focuses on bleach and includes a brief discussion of toners. We'll cover lightening with tint or color in Chapter 5.

The two main methods of lightening hair are solid color (all over) or dimensional color (frost or highlight). Many dimensional techniques such as foiling are, in my opinion, best left to the professional. If you have short hair, most retail stores offer frost kits that are easily mastered with practice or with help from a friend.

CAUTION: *I do not recommend frosting (pulling thru a cap) for long hair. It can be both painful and very difficult to achieve an even result.*

Although we will discuss the complete lightening process, the best results for lightening hair come from level changes of no more than three shades. Many colorists even feel that lightening no more than two shades from natural is best. The bigger the difference from the natural level, the more diligent you must be with upkeep.

The seven stages of lightening

Think back to the chapter on the color wheel. We talked about how brown hair is made of molecules from all three primary colors. For the sake of visualization, we said that it was made of one part blue, two parts red, and three parts yellow. When we use a bleach type of lightener, the molecules leave the hair in a dark to light order. When the hair starts to lighten, the blue molecules disappear first. Dark brown hair then takes on a red-brown tone as the blue molecules exit the hair. If we continue lightening, the next molecules leaving the hair are red. As color leaves the hair in stages, we are left with a continuing color change spectrum of red-orange, orange-red, orange-yellow or gold, yellow and ultimately pale yellow. We can only achieve pale yellow, if this is our goal, by having lightener with enough strength to lighten the number of levels we need. This will depend on our starting level. Also we must leave the lightener on for enough time to do the job.

CAUTION: If all the yellow is gone, we have hair that is white or without any pigment. This hair is considered over-lightened or over-processed hair. This is not a good thing. We can make pale yellow hair appear white with the use of a toner rather than over-lightening the hair. Currently the preference for blonde isn't the white blonde but fashion trends come and go so at some point it may be back in style.

The stages of lightening look like this:

Black - dark brown: Levels 1 - 3

Red-brown: Level 4

Red: Level 5

Red-orange: Level 6

Orange: Level 7

Gold: Level 8

Yellow: Level 9

Pale yellow: Level 10

White

These stages are the colors or the undertones you see as the hair gets progressively lighter, level by level. In other words, if you lighten brown Level 4 hair with bleach and you use a lightener with the strength to lighten two levels, you will have the red-orange undertone of a Level 6 as the dominant color left in the hair. Haven't we all known someone who used a Sun-In type product and ended up with orange hair? However, if our natural color is a Level 6 and we lighten two shades, we are left with a pretty gold Level 8 hair.

As you can see, success in lightening depends on figuring out what level of hair you are starting with, what level you want to be, and then making sure your product has the strength to lighten the correct number of levels. Also, make sure you read and follow the directions, and let the product process the correct amount of time.

Lightening with bleach will show up the undertone of the level to which you have chosen to lighten.

For example: You are a Level 4 and want to be a Level 8. To achieve this you can use a bleach that will lighten (or we say lift) four shades. When the bleach is done lifting the four shades, you will see a strong gold tone, the undertone of Level 8.

If gold or warm is not what you want to see, you can use a toner, a hair color product generally used to change the tone of hair that has been lightened. You would select a product with a base of blue-violet to minimize or counteract the gold. Using the toner will give you a neutral Level 8. Leave this blue-violet on the hair the full processing time and you could have an ash or drab Level 8. If gold is what you want to see, no toner is necessary and you are done coloring after the bleach has been rinsed and completely removed.

I must also add that many bleaches now contain drabbing agents to minimize the use of toners. The bleach lightens the hair but at the same time adds some blue or violet so the end result shows less of the undertone (which in our example is gold) resulting in a more neutral color.

Let's review the steps to basic bleaching.

1. Determine your natural or base level.

2. Decide the desired level.

3. Pick a product that can lift the desired number of levels.

4. Use a toner if necessary.

If you need to use a toner, you can choose from temporary, semi-permanent or a very mild permanent color. Remember, the hair is now porous from bleaching and will absorb the toner quickly. Choose the color you need to achieve your desired shade, a level no darker or possibly one shade lighter than your desired shade. In our example you would choose a toner with a blue-violet base in a Level 8 or 9.

Solid color bleaching

I can't leave the subject of lightening with bleach without a discussion of proper application. If you have chosen a solid color and are doing it on virgin hair, hair with no previous color, you will apply the bleach first to the cold shaft. The cold shaft is the hair that is ½ inch from the scalp and continues to the ends unless there is damaged or porous hair. If there is damage, the cold shaft ends where the damage or porosity begins. The hair that is porous absorbs color more quickly (Remember Chapter 2). Hair close to the scalp has body heat and lightens more quickly. That is why you begin applying your color ½ inch from the scalp and continue to the ends if the hair is healthy, or to the porous hair if the ends are damaged.

In our example where we are lightening four levels, we should apply bleach to the ends after the cold shaft has lightened one level if the damage is not too bad. If the ends are extremely porous, we should apply bleach to the ends after the cold shaft has lightened halfway or two shades. This is also the time to apply our product to the scalp. Make sure you have complete saturation on all hair at this time. When the bleach has lightened to the desired level, rinse and shampoo the lightener out completely or follow product directions. Failure to completely remove the entire product can result in scalp irritation.

If you are doing a retouch (just the roots) you must measure the length of new growth to be colored. If you are coloring a ½ inch regrowth, apply the bleach to the hair at the scalp and allow it to creep to the line of demarcation (the old color). If the regrowth is more than ½ inch, you must do the cold shaft of new growth before applying bleach to the scalp. The gold bands you've sometimes seen in blonde hair result when the regrowth was too long and the bleach was applied to the scalp at the same time as everything else. The scalp lightens faster and needs to be rinsed before the midsection was done.

In addition, remember that *bleach creeps*! (Great name for a band or maybe a bumper sticker.) If you apply the new bleach all the way to the line of the previously lightened hair, it will creep an additional ⅛ inch and you will cause further lightening to your previously lightened hair. This will make a brief section not only lighter but also more porous, causing toners to develop unevenly. Bleaching of previously bleached hair can cause breakage, so be careful. **Bleach creeps!!!!**

If you are going to get the full benefit from the lightening process you need to be diligent at keeping up with new growth. If you have a hard time with proper application, ask a friend or family member to help you, but make sure you adequately instruct them. Even better, have them read this chapter.

When the bleaching process is complete, you will want to see your color when it is dry before you decide on a toner. Wet bleached hair looks much more brassy or yellow than dry hair. Check before toning, particularly if this is the first bleaching experience for your hair. If you do decide to use a toner, remember Chapter 2 and our discussion of porosity:

If the ends seem damaged, apply from scalp to damage first and only to the ends as needed.

If this is a retouch, apply toner only where needed.

If your previously lightened hair still looks great, you may not have to tone it at all.

If it has gotten a little brassy, you can apply toner to the entire head.

Use your eyes, your judgment and the knowledge from Chapters 2 and 3 to make that determination. Make the decision on using a toner by judging the hair when it is dry.

One last reminder: Bleached hair is porous hair. If the ends have faded to very pale yellow and you put an ash toner on them, they will absorb that drab color and look dingy. Natural color has yellow, red and blue. The roots may need ash toner but the faded ends a little gold toner.

Use all your new hair color knowledge, and I know you will have beautiful results.

Dimensional color bleaching

Earlier I said that some techniques should be left to the professional. Foiling with bleach is one such technique. When you use a foil technique, you take specific strands, apply bleach and wrap the hair in foil to keep it separate from the other hair. If you do decide to foil with bleach, remember bleach's nasty little habit. Repeat after me: *Bleach creeps!!* It can expand and ooze out of the protective foil and make your hair a spotty mess. Foiling with bleach can be beautiful if done properly. When the hair being lightened is the desired color, pull the foils out of the hair and shampoo. If you need a toner for foiled hair, you should select a temporary or semi-permanent color. A permanent color toner is likely to affect the hair that has not been colored.

Frost kits are another great way to dimensionally color hair at home. You buy the kit which includes a cap or bonnet and a tool resembling a crochet hook. Place the cap on the head. Use the hook tool to pull selected strands through the cap. If you have very thin hair and pull lots of hair through the cap, you can look almost like you have a solid color. If you have very dense or thick hair and only pull a few hairs through the holes, you may not notice much highlight at all. Once you have pulled the desired amount of hair through, you will mix the lightener and apply it to all the hair evenly unless the ends are very porous. Follow the directions for processing time but also watch the lightening process to determine when rinsing and shampooing should take place. If you decide to use a toner, you can even use a permanent color if you leave the cap on while toning. If you decide to tone with the cap off, a temporary or semi-permanent toner is best. This will leave the uncolored hair without noticeable change.

Hair painting and scrunching the ends with bleach are other techniques used for dimensional color results. If you choose to use these techniques, remember undertones. Bleach has to completely penetrate to properly do its job. If penetration is not complete you may not lighten to your desired level. Orange or brassy hair is the result particularly if you are starting with hair that is Level 6 or lower. The techniques themselves are simple—just put the bleach where you want to lighten while keeping it off the rest of the hair. Watch the color development; shampoo when the hair has lightened to your satisfaction.

Being blond

I love blonde hair. I love highlighted hair also. The products that are available today can make almost any base color into blonde. However, just because you *can* be a blonde doesn't mean you *should* be a blonde. All blonde is not pretty blonde, but if you are going to get pleasure from a change to blonde, go for it. Have fun with your hair color.

Remember, the more levels of change you make, the faster the regrowth shows. Be diligent in maintaining your new color. Take care of the darker regrowth. You want to get noticed but hopefully not for your roots.

Closing thoughts

Bleach doesn't have to be scary. Here is bleaching wisdom in a nutshell:

- Determine your natural shade; decide your desired shade, and shop for a product that can do the job.

- Keep in mind the undertone that will be dominant when you lighten to your desired shade. A toner might be necessary.

- Bleach creeps!

- Pale yellow hair will grab whatever base color is in your toner.

- Dark roots with blonde ends look tacky.

There. You've got it. Happy bleaching.

Chapter 5
Lightening hair with color

Many experts believe you should not lighten your natural hair color more than two shades. If this amount of lightening is your desire, it can be done with color rather than bleach. When I learned about color in beauty school many years ago, the following information was not taught. I don't know if the permanent color products were not perfected to the current level or if it just was not taught. The beauty of lightening with color is that you can lighten and tone in one step. The only drawback to lightening with color is that you usually cannot make the drastic changes that are possible with bleach.

> *Color will not lift color.*

The information in this chapter concerning lightening with color applies only to virgin hair. Virgin hair means hair with no previous artificial color. If you are trying to lighten hair that has been previously colored, you must use bleach to make any significant change. Tint will not lift tint. Let me say this again: Color will not lift color. Attempting to lighten a color that came out too dark with another box of lighter color doesn't work. Bleach or color removers are the only ways to lighten unsatisfactory color.

The rules for lightening with color

As we discussed in Chapter 1, permanent color is the only color that will lighten hair. There is a simple formula that helps us decide which box of permanent color to buy:

$$D \times 2 - B = F$$

Let's decode the formula to see how we can easily choose a permanent color to lighten the hair.

D = **Desired shade** or the color we want

B = **Base color** or natural color.

F = **Formula**, the number on the box of color we will select or the level of color we use to do our lightening.

To apply the formula we multiply our desired shade by 2 and subtract the level of our base color. The result (F) is the level of color we should purchase. This formula is designed to work with color that uses 20 volume peroxide.

The formula doesn't tell us what tone of color to buy but we can figure that out by referring back to our chart of undertones. (Please note that for lightening purposes, if our natural level or base color is between two shades, use the darker shade to plug into the formula). For example, if you are between a 5 or a 6, choose Level 5 to use with the formula.

Let's say that we are a Level 5 and want to be a Level 7. We put those numbers into the formula and it looks like this:

$$7 \times 2 - 5 = 9$$

We multiply our desired level (7) by 2 and subtract the level of our base color (5) resulting in 9, the color level of the product we need to purchase.

If we refer back to our undertone chart we see that the dominant color or undertone when we lighten to a Level 7 is orange. If we want to have an orange Level 7 as the

> *If you are lightening hair with color, you should almost always use ash.*

desired shade we would buy a Level 9 with a neutral base. Then when we lighten we will get the undertone that happens naturally, which is orange. If we don't want orange we will choose a color that has a base that will counteract orange. By referring to the color wheel we know that the color to neutralize orange is blue, which is ash. Therefore, we will buy a box of Level 9 color with an ash or blue base to get the Level 5 hair lightened to a Level 7 without being too brassy.

Once you are used to using the formula and the habit of referring back to the color wheel, lightening with color will be a breeze. The D or desired shade is what you want. The B or base is what you have. The F is the formula or the color you should purchase after you have checked out the undertones.

Keep in mind that most colors purchased for lightening purposes are ash shades. The obvious reason is that we don't want brassy hair from the undertones. Also know that many color companies' lightest box available for home use is a Level 10. This limits how drastic a change we can attempt.

Note the following example:

8 x 2 - 4 = 12

This is a Level 4 that wants to be a Level 8. If there is no box of color that is equal to a 12, you can't lighten with color. You must use bleach to get to a Level 8.

Professional cosmetologists have broader color options and stronger peroxide which are not available to most home colorists. Therefore, you are somewhat limited if you wish to use color to change your hair greater than a couple levels.

You can use this formula always to see if lightening with color is a possibility for you. Also you can use all the same techniques for lightening with color that you use for lightening with bleach. The best part is that most color doesn't creep and you can have a one step process, no toning necessary.

Lightening significantly gray hair with color

In Chapter 2 when we talked about levels, you will remember that we called white hair a Level 11 with no pigment. If we are lightening hair with bleach, obviously the white hairs will stay white. If we are lightening a head with color, the white hairs will become the color that we have chosen for our formula. Let's take a look at how this works using our original example but adding 10% white hair.

$$D \times 2 - B = F$$

$$7 \times 2 - 5 = 9$$

If 10% of the hair is white or a Level 11 and we are using a color that is a Level 9, that means that 90% of the hair will be a Level 7 and 10% of the hair will be a Level 9. The white hair will be darker and the dark hair will be lighter.

It's always the big picture that is our first concern rather than each individual hair strand. If we decide to use a Level 9 ash, we have to consider the effect it will have on the white hair. If the white is all around the face, it might look a little drab and we may need to reevaluate. An ash shade around the face may not be appropriate. If the white is scattered throughout the head, the ash will be insignificant on the white and may be necessary to take care of the undertone when lifting to a Level 7. If we look back to Chapter 3 we will remember that white hair has no yellow, no red and no blue. Our percentage of white and its placement will determine if we do a little customizing to keep the skin tones looking nice with the hair color. If the majority of white is around the face, we could use 9 neutral or warm around the face and 9 ash on the rest.

People who have colored for years may not realize how much whiter they are now compared to when they started coloring. This is the reason many become dissatisfied with a color they have used for years. The absence of warmth brought on by the progression of white can make a color that was once satisfactory feel and look washed out.

Let's consider the same example but with 50% gray that is fairly even throughout the head. If we use an ash Level 9, 50% of our hairs become an ash Level 9 and 50% of our hairs are lifted to a Level 7, with the orange undertone cancelled.

If we look at the finished hair, the big picture, we can determine if it has enough warmth to look pretty. If the hair seems too drab, it is time to switch to a neutral color. My general recommendation is that if there is 50% or more white hair, it is time to use less ash and a more neutral color. You may get warmth from the hair that is being lightened but the overall hair will be prettier if the 50% white hair is a neutral color rather than ash.

Our last example will be on a head that is mostly white. If the dark hair is minimal, you should most likely use the color you want to be and only briefly consider the effects brought on by the dark hair becoming lighter. Although you must consider skin tone and personal preference, I tend to use warmer colors on clients who are mostly white. I recommend that you choose warm colors also. This subject will be covered thoroughly in the next chapter.

Summary of lightening gray hair

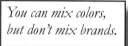

You can mix colors, but don't mix brands.

Although individual preferences need to be considered, the following is a guide for quick selection. If your desired result is a neutral, natural looking color and you are lightening the hair with color, use ash for heads up to 50 % gray, use a neutral color for 51% to 75% gray and consider a warm color for more than 75%. Remember, this is a guide only. Never underestimate your judgment or substitute my opinion for yours. Also, don't hesitate to mix two colors together or to customize. One color around the face and another for the rest of the head is often a great option.

If you decide to mix shades, be sure to stay within the same brand. Also choose the brand of color that is easiest to figure out. Many companies have already numbered their home color products with the system I have described, Levels 1 thru 10, but may use another number that signifies the tone. Definitely get help from a clerk or an 800 number if the system is unclear.

The details make the difference
When you are using color to lighten hair and doing a retouch, do not feel you must pull the color thru the ends. If the ends are already light, why create more porosity. If you need to drab some brassy ends, add some shampoo or conditioner to your ash color before you pull the color thru the ends for the last few minutes. Do the same with a warm color for ends that are faded too light or white.

Also know that the professional colorist has all types of concentrates to drab or warm any color, conditioners to equalize porosity, and different volumes of peroxide for more or less lift. If you have read and applied this information and still can't get a color you are happy with, don't hesitate to ask your stylist for suggestions.

Review of the process
Step 1 - What I have—My natural level or base level. *It must be virgin hair.*

Step 2 - What I want—My desired level

Step 3 - The formula

Step 4 - The tone or the undertone—Do I want it or do I need to neutralize or counteract it?

Step 5 - The technique—Solid or dimensional?

Step 6 - When in doubt, do a test strand. Mix a small amount of the color and apply it to hair that won't be seen easily. When in doubt, test it out!

Closing thoughts

Lightening with color is faster and generally less damaging than lightening with bleach. Also, color doesn't creep like bleach. You can't get the levels of lift that you can with bleach, but for many that is not the goal. Use the information in this chapter if it is applicable for your hair and your desired shade, but if you are tired of light hair and are thinking about going darker, go to Chapter 6.

Chapter 6
Deepening your shade

Let's be honest. If you have reached a certain level of maturity, you probably shouldn't strive to have hair as dark as you had when you were in your twenties. It makes most of us look too harsh and our friends talk about us behind our backs, accusing us of trying too hard to look young again. If you are still young, you can do the Elvira thing and get away with it. Our skin tones change with age along with our hair. Therefore, to achieve the most flattering color you should strive to be age-appropriate when choosing among the deeper shades.

Darkening your shade is easy for most heads. The usual system is to find your natural shade, decide what shade you want to be and use that color. It can be that simple. However, my job is to get you beautiful results so we will discuss the finer points. If you can't decide your natural level and are trying to choose between two, choose the lighter level when you contemplate going darker. You can always go darker later but if you pick a color too dark to begin with, it is harder to lighten back up.

Going darker — Why?
A major portion of the color market for darker hair is the cover-the-gray group. As we suggested in the previous chapter, they may not want their pigmented hair darker but do want the Level 11 white hairs colored.

37

Another group of color customers who choose to go darker are made up of those who have previously had highlights or lighter hair and now want to go back to their natural color. Some of this lightening could simply have been the result of being sun bleached or chemically damaged. Hair, particularly the ends, can also lighten from perms or relaxers.

The last reason to go darker, and the most prevalent reason for the younger crowd, is just because they feel like it. It can be fun to be different, to be deep red one month and black the next. Change is good and although it is not always our best look, it does create attention and gets us noticed.

Going darker — How?
In the beginning of this book we discussed the types of hair colors: temporary, semi- or demi-permanent, and permanent color. The first three are great ways to go darker with less commitment. Let's discuss how they are best used.

Temporary color such as a color rinse works great for hair that has a small amount of gray that you would like to camouflage. If you regularly color your hair with semi-permanent or permanent color, temporary color is a good backup to use to cover regrowth or refresh faded ends between color applications. Also temporary color works great to deepen faded color after a perm.

There are currently some very bright temporary colors on the market that make a subtle change to pigmented or natural hair but become loud, screaming colors when applied to pre-lightened hair. Not much more needs to be said about temporary colors except to remind you to follow manufacturers' instructions. And remember that pre-lightened hair can grab temporary color. If your hair is bleached out, be a little cautious.

Semi-permanent color is also known as "deposit only" color. It can be a great choice for darker hair if you do not have a high percentage of gray. You can change your color with very little damage to the hair. You can also protect previously damaged, lightened or faded ends by using semi-permanent color. By following manufacturer's instructions carefully, you can even dimensionally color hair with semi-permanent color. Making only some hair darker is called "low-lighting."

Choosing a color when you are going darker with semi-permanent is very easy. Find your natural level, find your desired color and use it.

There are a few things to remember. Fine hair will look darker than coarse hair even if you have the same base level and choose the same box of color. If your hair is fine, you may want to

Unless you are following a fad, ends that are darker than the rest of the hair aren't natural looking.

choose a lighter color than you first thought. You can always recolor a darker shade if it is not dark enough easier than you can lighten up color that is too dark.

If you apply color to the entire head, which is the norm for semi-permanent color, the hair will generally be the same color from scalp to ends. This is important to note because natural hair is always slightly lighter at the ends, particularly if the hair has any length to it. Check and see, but I would bet that if you have hair four inches or longer that is not colored, you will find a slight variance in the end color compared to the roots. My reason for mentioning this is that dark ends usually give a harder appearance to the face. If this is of concern, follow your own judgment. If you feel color on the ends is necessary, you may not want to process the ends for the entire time.

Remember also that semi-permanent color can begin fading with the first shampoo. Always check the color once it has dried. Wet hair looks darker than dry hair. If it is too dark from the start, start shampooing with a fairly strong shampoo.

My best recommendation is that if you are in doubt about color selection, choose the lighter shade. You can always go darker later. It seems a waste to try to fade a new color right from the start.

Final note: Reds fade the fastest of any color. This seems to be true of both semi- and permanent color.

Going darker on gray hair

Semi-permanent color is a great choice for covering gray if the gray is not dominant. It is a great starter color. Remember in a previous chapter where we talked about the big picture? Well, if you have had gray hair for any length of time, you have been looking at a big picture that is lighter than it was when you weren't gray. If you use color the same as your natural and all that hair is dark again, the big picture will be much darker than you have been used to seeing. If that is what you want, great, but a better choice might be to choose a couple shades lighter than your natural. The natural color will not change but the gray hair will take on a softer highlighted look. It can be very pretty. Also remember that if you do have white hair, it has no pigment and can take on the appearance of the base color. A beautiful red can look awesome when applied to brown hair and hideous when applied to white hair. Remember, natural looking hair has some of all the primary colors. If you only add red pigment to white hair it will not look as natural because it is missing some primany colors. A few white hairs colored red blend in, but a significant number will usually be too intense. If that is not your intention, choose a color that has brown with some red, or color the hair blonde or brown first to cover the gray and then color with red for brightness. You can easily do this type of coloring with semi-permanent or demi-permanent color.

Going darker on prelightened hair

Remember the color wheel? If your hair has been previously lightened to a Level 8 or above, it is devoid of all blue primary color, most if not all red primary color, and possibly some yellow primary color. If you decide to go back to your natural level, you must choose a color that has red and yellow to restore those primary colors to the hair.

If you color back with a neutral color or an ash color, your ends can end up looking gray, green or muddy. Those missing primary colors need to be replaced. Some colorists use color fillers, or they color bleached out hair with a red-gold color first to fill in the missing pigment and then color again with the desired shade of brown. This can get complicated; don't hesitate to contact a professional for color correction.

If your lightened hair is not that drastic, you can usually just use the desired shade and have great results. Just remember to consider your hair's porosity to determine processing time. Porous hair absorbs color faster and it fades faster. Sometimes reconditioning is in order before and after the color service.

Also, there are lots of products with sunscreen to keep the fading to a minimum.

Going darker with permanent color

The guidelines we discussed for making hair darker with semi-permanent color apply in many ways to permanent color. One big difference is that with permanent color you can get 100% gray coverage. Many color companies recommend using permanent color if you need to color hair that is at least 30% gray. Another difference is that with 20 volume peroxide you can also lighten the darker hair while making the white hair darker.

Keep in mind that texture is very important with permanent color. Fine hair can look up to two shades darker than coarse hair using the same hair color and starting with the same original level of color. I recommend choosing a shade one or two shades lighter for fine hair.

You must also consider porosity. If the ends are damaged, either recondition them before the color service or adjust your timing. If you are doing a retouch (the new growth) and the ends are good, just color the regrowth. If the ends are slightly faded, pull the color through the ends for just the last five or ten minutes.

The big picture when going darker

We have talked about the big picture several times in previous chapters. When we are coloring gray hair darker with permanent color, we need to decide if we want all the hair darker or just the gray hair darker. If we color the gray hair to match the pigmented hair, the big picture will be much darker than you have been accustomed to seeing. If this is your goal, go for it always considering both texture and porosity in your color choice. If you don't necessarily want the big picture to be that much darker, here are some options from which to choose.

Option 1 - Low-light the hair. You can use a frost cap, foil or a painting technique to darken only some of the hairs. This will leave some gray hair which makes the big picture lighter than if all the hair were colored as dark as your natural color. This low-lighting is great for easing your way into color. It many times takes your hair back to a time when there wasn't as much gray. Low-lighting also works great for blonde hair that has faded ends. In this low-lighting situation always remember to supply the missing primary color.

Option 2 - Color the gray hair darker while lifting the natural hair a shade or two. This will result in a big picture that is not much darker overall.

The instructions for this procedure are in Chapter 5 - Lightening Hair with Color, but let's do a quick review.

Find your natural level and your percentage of white.

Decide on your desired shade and use the formula to figure out the end result. The percentage of gray and the undertone that will show up when you lighten the pigmented hair will determine the tone you will use.

Here's an example: If you are a natural Level 5 with 40% gray, a solid Level 5 may be too dark for your current skin tone. You decide you could live with an overall Level 7. To make white hair a Level 7 you use a 7 or an 8 if the hair is fine. To make a Level 5 into a Level 7 you use a Level 9.

Remember the formula 7 x 2 - 5 = 9. Now you must decide between a Level 7, Level 8 or Level 9, or a combination of two shades. Your decision will be based on texture of hair and personal preference. Ask yourself if you would rather be lighter or darker. The tone you use will be determined by the undertone present when you lift dark hair, your own skin tone and preference and by the percentage of white. Generally speaking, the more white hair you have, the more you should lean to neutral or warm tones. The more pigmented hair you have, the more often you should use an ash shade to counteract the undertones, thereby keeping the big picture from being too brassy.

Option 3 - Deposit color and highlight during the same color service. It's a fairly new option. Many color companies are coming out with prepackaged kits to accomplish both processes. You would color the hair all over first and then go back and paint some highlights after the first color is rinsed. The finished look is lighter and generally softer looking than a solid color. The highlights are usually around the face or thru the top. This gives a youthful appearance. You can use the same technique but with bolder colors or chunkier sections for a more radical look.

Remember: if you don't buy a kit that comes with both deposit color and highlights, you must use bleach to achieve any noticeable lift on previously colored hair. Tint/color will not lift tint.

Closing thoughts

Natural hair is usually lighter at the ends, especially if your hair is long.

Dimensional color looks more natural.

Look at and study the hair colors you see before you decide if you want to have darker hair.

If you get your hair too dark for your liking, it can be hard to lighten it back up without significant damage with at-home products. You may require professional help.

You are never too old to color your hair. My oldest hair color client was 101.

Avoid getting tied to the idea that if you were a Level 4 in your twenties that you must be a Level 4 in your forties, fifties and beyond.

Chapter 7
Changing color while staying the same level

The information you see in this chapter is very similar to Chapter 6. You can use temporary, semi-permanent, demi-permanent or permanent color to achieve a color that is the same level but a different tone or to make the white hair the same color as the pigmented hair. As always, if you have to choose between two levels to match your base color, choose the lighter level. This rule of thumb will save you from getting hair color results that are too dark.

If gray coverage is your goal and you have less than 30% gray, I highly recommend semi-permanent color. I also recommend semi-permanent color as a toner for hair that has been bleached.

While keeping in mind your hair's texture and porosity, you may find the table below a useful guide for semi-permanent color.

Desired result	The choice
Brighten color	2 levels lighter
Blend gray	1 level lighter
Cover gray completely	Desired level
Refresh color faded from sun, perm or relaxer	1 level lighter
Tone bleached hair	1 level lighter

While I don't always recommend a chart as a substitute for your judgment, this one is pretty easy to use if you should need some extra help.

Toning bleached hair

Imagine that you have pulled your hair through a frost cap and lightened it to a Level 8. The hair is light enough but too gold and you would like to change the tone of the hair to minimize the gold. What should you do? There are a variety of choices. We will cover several in this section.

If you have a temporary color shampoo on hand, that may be all that is necessary. Many shampoos and some conditioners are available with a violet base which will counteract the gold. Once applied, the product's violet base will make the gold hair appear more neutral and less brassy.

When you use any toner, watch your hair ends. If the ends are not gold because they are more porous, the ends may grab the base, which is violet, and look gray. If these ends are lighter and need little or no color correction (toning), put regular shampoo or conditioner in them before toning to keep absorption to a minimum.

I have a personal preference for semi-permanent toners. You can choose a level, a tone or mix a couple together to customize the color. You can also apply the toner to the entire head without fear of changing (lightening) the unbleached hair.

Remember that bleached hair is damaged or porous hair.

Watch your ends because they may not need toner for the full processing time if at all.

Here's an example: Using the chart on the previous page as a guide, you'll see that if you wanted to tone your Level 8 bleached hair to neutralize the brassy gold, you would use a Level 9 color with a violet base. If the ends aren't brassy, don't apply toner.

Permanent color can tone bleached hair in the same way that semi-permanent color does. The difference is that you can't use permanent color on unbleached hair without changing it. The permanent color would cause some lightening. If the whole head has been bleached, feel free to use permanent color as a toner. If you are using a frost cap, you can tone with permanent color before you remove the cap. If you are using foils, it is almost impossible to tone hair with permanent color. Using a Level 9 permanent color toner will lighten the virgin hair as it tones the bleached hair. Unless you don't mind the rest of the hair being lighter, skip the toning with permanent color.

Red

I can't end this chapter without mentioning red, a very big segment of the color market. Beautiful reds are not always easy to achieve and are hard to keep. They seem to fade faster than any other color unless, of course, you want them to fade. If you are new to hair color or are considering red for the first time, I recommend a semi-permanent color. Keep in mind that there are blue/reds, true reds, orange/reds, as well as red/ brown and don't forget copper and strawberry blonde. Choose your desired level and desired tone based on your skin tone.

If you have gray hair, remember the gray will show the base color strongly. A brown with some red may be a better choice than red with little or no brown. You may even want to color your gray the same as your natural color and then apply another color with red to prevent the white hair from being too vibrant.

If you are positive that you want to be a redhead, permanent color is a very practical choice. If you are a natural Level 6 or darker, remember that you can get a little red undertone from the lifting action of permanent color. This gives you a much wider range of choices than you can achieve with semi-permanent color because red can come from lifting your natural color as well as from pigment in the bottle.

Closing thoughts

Products are available for you to be almost any color you want to be. Learn the whole system of color and you can achieve any result. Just remember, if you have to choose between two colors to determine your base color, pick the lighter color.

If you are not sure which color product to choose, pick the lighter. It is easier to color again darker than to try to lighten up newly processed color.

Also remember that the ends on unprocessed hair are naturally lighter than the hair at the scalp. You must analyze and decide the effect you want with your new color.

Chapter 8
How to apply color

You have analyzed your hair, decided what you want and bought the box or bottles of color. Now what?

In this chapter we will briefly discuss the application of color. Use this as a guide, but also follow your manufacturer's instructions. Read the directions first because some colors ask you to do a patch test before applying the color. This is a test where you mix a little of the color you plan to use and apply it to the skin in an inconspicuous place such as behind your ear. If the skin gets red or itchy or painful, you may be allergic to that color and should not use it.

Solid color

Depending on the product you choose, your application may be poured from a bottle, applied with a brush from a bowl, or even sprayed from a can. Whatever method you use to apply the product, the goal is complete coverage.

If you are coloring the whole head, start by dividing the head into four sections. Do this by making one part from ear to ear and another part from the front, center forehead to the rear, center nape. Clip these sections.

Start the application in the upper portion of one of the four sections. If you are using color, use ½-inch sections. If you are bleaching, use ¼-inch partings or sections.

If this is a virgin application, you apply color from scalp to ends except in the case of extremely porous ends.

When you're using bleach or lightening with color, apply the product to the cold shaft first. (The cold shaft, remember, is the hair that is ½-inch from the scalp and continues to the ends unless there is damaged or porous hair.) Work quickly and begin your timing when all the hair you intend to color is saturated. If lightening, pull the product thru the ends and apply to the scalp only after the cold shaft is partially processed. Rinse when you have the desired results and shampoo the remaining color out of the hair.

If you are attempting a solid color with permanent color to new growth only, do not mix the entire contents of each bottle. You can save the unmixed portions of product to use another time. When the timing on the new growth is complete, you can pull color thru a few strands to blend before you rinse.

Dimensional color

If you're using a frost cap, comb your hair the direction you style it before putting on the frost cap. Pull small pieces of hair out through the holes in the cap with your hook. The more holes you use, the more colored hair you will have. Try not to pull through big hunks of hair unless you are looking for a very chunky outcome. I find subtle to be better, but the choice is yours.

You can also use a paint brush to randomly stroke color onto the hair. This is called "balayage." You must be careful with this technique because you can end up with a mess. If you do choose this technique, remember that it is most often used for a change of no more than two levels.

You can accomplish foil highlighting or low-lighting by isolating selected strands, applying color and wrapping them in protective foil. This technique takes time and practice and should probably be done by experienced hands. If you are going to attempt it, work quickly. Don't use chunky sections of hair unless you are sure it will give you the result you want.

Other techniques

Keep your eyes open for the newest color techniques in fashion magazines. Styles and trends change quickly and you never know when you will run across a new look to try with color.

Closing thoughts

Not every home colorist can master all the techniques discussed in this chapter. If you are going to attempt more than a solid color, practice your application with conditioner to build your speed and confidence. Better yet, ask a family member or friend for help.

Chapter 9
Final thoughts

This is the end of this book but hopefully just the beginning of your fun with hair color. I hope this information will bring you some confidence when you choose color to apply at home. If you master this information, you will be able to use it for many years to come.

Don't forget that most hair color companies have 800 numbers, so don't hesitate to contact them directly if you have a question or problem.

When you shop for color, buy the product that is easiest for you to select the proper level and tone. A beautiful picture on a box or a great commercial means nothing if you cannot determine which product will give you the result you want. You must know if your product is permanent, semi-permanent, or temporary. If you can't tell, keep shopping until you find a product you are sure about. You must know what level you are starting with and what level you wish to achieve.

Also remember that any mistake can eventually be fixed, but it may take a professional to properly correct a color mistake. However, the better you understand the information in this book, the less likely you will ever make a color mistake.

Just for fun, go to the color aisle in a store; watch and listen to the people who are shopping. A frightening number of them haven't a clue about which box to choose. Now that you have finished this book, you won't be one of the clueless. You can determine your starting level, your desired level, and what type of product you need to purchase to reach the hair color you desire. Read the labels and you'll never again have to guess what product to purchase. You can relax and have fun creating new color and a new look for yourself.

Happy coloring!!

Glossary

Chemical process - Any change made to hair with chemicals including perm solution, relaxer or hair color. These chemicals can change the strength and condition of the hair.

Cold shaft - Hair starting ½-inch from the scalp to the ends or to where major damage is present in the ends.

Color - Word used interchangeably to mean actual color of hair or the product to be applied.

Conditioner - A product that coats the outside of the hairshaft making the hair less tangled and feel as if it is less damaged.

Drab - A word used by colorists which describes either the ash tones or the color that appears when a color that is too ash is used on hair. It means without warmth. If the hair is too gold or warm, we use an ash tone to try to drab out the warmth. Drabbing tones have a base of either violet, blue or green.

Level - A word used by cosmetologists to describe the lightness or darkness of hair. Level 1 is the darkest and Level 10 is the lightest blonde. For training purposes we describe white hair as Level 11.

Line of demarcation - Where virgin hair meets previously colored hair.

Porosity - The ability of the hair to absorb moisture. Damaged hair absorbs moisture (color) quickly. Damaged or porous hair can also fade rapidly. This is important to know to help determine processing time or to delay coloring until the hair has been reconditioned.

Reconditioner - A product that can penetrate inside the hair shaft to make hair stronger and less damaged.

Tint - A word used interchangeably to mean either the process of coloring or the color product.

Tone - Refers to the warmth or coolness of a color. For example: Medium brown hair could be red brown, golden brown, ash brown or neutral.

Toner - Another word that describes a hair color product. The product is generally used to change the tone of hair that has been lightened but is not the shade or tone that you desire. They can be any color that will do the job, but the name "Toner" is usually seen only in the products available to professionals.

Virgin hair - Hair that has never been colored.